YOUR KNOWLEDGE HAS VALUE

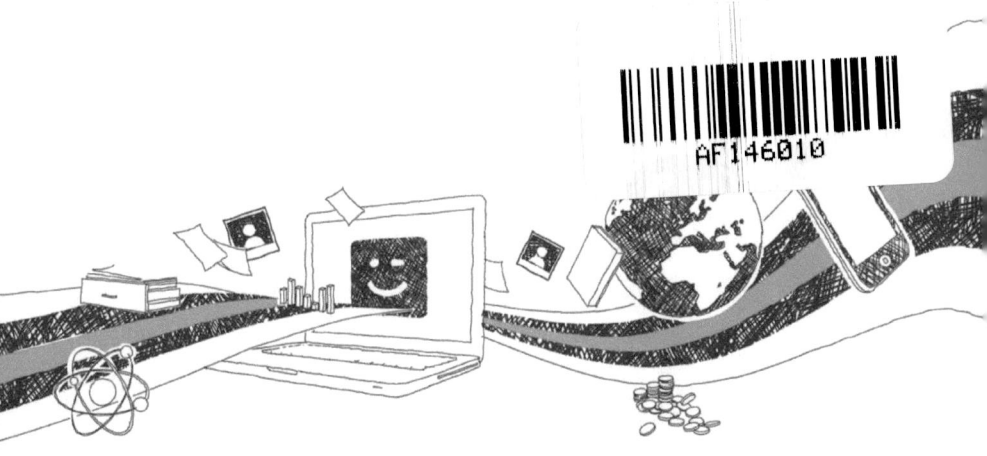

AF146010

- We will publish your bachelor's and
  master's thesis, essays and papers

- Your own eBook and book -
  sold worldwide in all relevant shops

- Earn money with each sale

Upload your text at www.GRIN.com
and publish for free

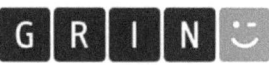

Imprint:

Copyright © 2019 GRIN Verlag
Print and binding: Books on Demand GmbH, Norderstedt Germany
ISBN: 9783668957336

This book at GRIN:

https://www.grin.com/document/470279

Xue Mi

The Relationship among Governance Structure, R & D Investment and Performance of Pharmaceutical Enterprises

GRIN Verlag

GRIN - Your knowledge has value

Since its foundation in 1998, GRIN has specialized in publishing academic texts by students, college teachers and other academics as e-book and printed book. The website www.grin.com is an ideal platform for presenting term papers, final papers, scientific essays, dissertations and specialist books.

Visit us on the internet:

http://www.grin.com/

http://www.facebook.com/grincom

http://www.twitter.com/grin_com

Research on the relationship among Governance structure, R & D Investment and performance of Pharmaceutical Enterprises

Xue Mi

Department of International Pharmaceutical Business,

China Pharmaceutical University, Nanjing, Jiangsu, China

Abstract: Objective: To study the relationship between the governance structure and the input intensity of R & D investment of pharmaceutical enterprises, and to check the lag effect of R & D input on the performance. Methods: The data of the balanced panel of 133 medical-listed enterprises from 2009 to 2016 were taking as samples, the regression analysis was performed by using the STATA13.0 software. Results: In the aspect of the ownership structure, the state-owned control has a negative effect on the R & D investment intensity, and the equity concentration degree and the equity balance degree are positive. In terms of the governance of the board of directors, the proportion of the two-level and independent directors is positively affecting the strength of R & D and the scale of the board of directors has a negative effect. In that case of executive motivation, the share power incentive and salary incentive do not play the desired positive role. The lag effect of R & D investment on enterprise performance has verified. With the passage of time, the relationship between R & D investment and enterprise performance has gradually changed from significant negative to significant positive. Conclusion: Based on the research results, some suggestions are put forward to provide empirical evidence for optimizing the internal governance structure of pharmaceutical enterprises and improving the efficiency of R & D.

Keywords: Pharmaceutical enterprises; Corporate governance; Investment in R & D; Enterprise performance; Hysteresis effect

Table of Contents

1. Foreword

Pharmaceutical industry is a high-tech industry, listed by the state as a strategic emerging industry and the "made in China 2025" key development areas. The 13th five-year Plan of the pharmaceutical industry focuses on promoting innovation, pointing out that in order to realize the upgrading and development of the pharmaceutical industry during the 13th five-year Plan, the key is to implement the innovation-driven development strategy, and innovation must be placed at the core of the overall development of the pharmaceutical industry. Strengthen the technical strength as the strategic fulcrum of building a powerful pharmaceutical country; strengthen the innovation ability of pharmaceutical industry [1]. Under this background, the majority of pharmaceutical enterprises should make great efforts to perfect the innovation mechanism of enterprise-oriented, market-oriented, industry-university-research combination, and grasp the opportunity, increase R & D investment, speed up the pace of innovation.

In order to deal with the complex and changeable industry environment and stand out from the fierce industry competition, pharmaceutical enterprises not only need to pay attention to technological innovation and R & D investment, but also need to improve the internal governance structure of the company. The corporate governance structure refers to the structural institutional arrangement in order to achieve the best operating performance of the company, and the corporate ownership and management rights are based on trust responsibility to form mutual checks and balances. Therefore, the corporate governance structure affects the decision-making of technological innovation, then affects the efficiency of R & D investment and innovation activities, and finally affects the performance of enterprises [2]. However, due to the professional nature of the business content of pharmaceutical enterprises, the current chairperson and general manager and other business executives are all the internal governance structure of the company adjusted and optimized by professional managers. Therefore, there is stillroom for improvement of the internal governance structure of the current enterprise.

3

Taking pharmaceutical listed enterprises as research samples, this paper studies the influence of each variable of corporate governance structure on the intensity of R & D investment, and tests the lag effect of R & D investment on enterprise performance by using the method of empirical analysis. In order to optimize the internal governance structure of pharmaceutical enterprises and improve the efficiency of innovation research and develop to provide empirical evidence.

2. Literature review and hypothetical development

2.1 Corporate governance structure and R & D investment intensity

Review the relevant literature (Xiang Chaojin et al., 2003 [3],Zhou Jian et al., 2012[4],Lu Tong et al., 2014[5],Chen Lilin et al., 2015 [6],Ye Chen Gang et al., 2016 [7],Feng Taozhu et al., 2017 [8],Zhang Min et al., 2017[9],Xie Haijuan et al., 2018 [10]), Most of them choose different indicators to measure corporate governance structure from three aspects: equity structure, board governance and executive incentive. This article selects the nature of equity, equity concentration, equity balance on behalf of the ownership structure; the size of the board of directors, the proportion of independent directors, the establishment of two positions to represent the board of directors Governance; executive equity incentives and executive compensation incentives represent executive incentives. Strive to build more perfect corporate governance structure variables.

2.1.1 Nature of stock rights

The state-owned enterprises are controlled by the state, their business objectives are diversified and restricted by many non-economic objectives, the motivation of technological innovation is greatly weakened, the subject of property rights is false, the subject of interest is vague, and it is difficult to focus on the long-term development of the enterprise. Because of the multi-layer principal-agent relationship, it is difficult to form an effective supervision mechanism, and it is easy to form the insider control, thus avoiding the risk. Reduce investment in innovation. Kornai et al., think that budget soft constraints will restrain the enthusiasm of managers of state-owned enterprises to carry out efficient operation and management of enterprises [11]. Zhang Qixiu pointed out that the state's informal intervention in state-owned enterprises will have a negative impact on the business decision-making and strategic implementation of the enterprises. It will also damage R & D investment conversion efficiency [12]. Many scholars have shown that state-owned holding companies have little investment in innovation and lack of efficiency compared to private property holding companies [13]. Based on this, this paper proposes the following assumptions:

5

H1：State-owned holding has a negative impact on the intensity of R & D investment.

2.1.2 Equity concentration

Moderate concentration of equity is beneficial to technological innovation of enterprises. Major shareholders pay attention to the long-term stable development of enterprises, and have the ability and motivation to take risks, so they can effectively stimulate and monitor the technological innovation activities of enterprises, increase R & D investment in order to obtain high returns and the long-term profitability of enterprises. In addition, minority shareholders pay more attention to short-term returns; there are speculation and "free ride" behavior. Based on this, this paper proposes the following assumptions:

H2：Equity concentration has a positive impact on the intensity of R & D investment.

2.1.3 Equity balance degree

The mechanism of stockholding checks and balances means that many large shareholders control each other, restrain and supervise each other, share the control and decision-making power of the company together, and avoid "one share being the only big one". Equity checks and balances are beneficial to reduce agency conflicts, restrict the behavior of large shareholders encroaching on the interests of small and medium shareholders, and make management decision-making accord with the maximization of enterprise value. It is beneficial to restrain insider control, to form a good internal governance mechanism, to improve the scientific nature of business decision-making, to carry out R & D activities, and to realize the long-term objectives of enterprises. Based on this, this paper proposes the following assumptions:

H3：Equity balance degree has a positive impact on R & D investment intensity.

2.1.4 Board size

The board of directors is the main decision-maker in business activities [2], therefore, it also plays an important role in setting R & D investment. The expansion of the board of directors can bring in more experts from different academic backgrounds and working experiences to improve the scientific nature of decision-making, but at the same time it will also result in a decline in the efficiency of communication among members and even a "free ride" phenomenon [14]. It is not conducive to the rapid and efficient decision-making in the competitive market, thus reducing the innovation efficiency and R & D intensity. Based on this, this paper proposes the following assumptions:

H4: Board size has a negative impact on R & D investment intensity.

2.1.5 Proportion of independent directors

Independent directors have different professional backgrounds and skills experience, reflect the voices from the outside world, can broaden the vision of internal directors, improve the quality of innovation decision-making, effectively deal with the uncertainty in the external environment, and promote innovation and change. Many scholars have shown that the investment level of innovation R & D in enterprises with higher proportion of independent directors is significantly higher than that of enterprises with lower proportion of independent directors [15]. Based on this, this paper proposes the following assumptions:

H5: The proportion of independent directors has a positive effect on R & D investment intensity.

2.1.6 two-job setup

The principal-agent theory plays a dominant role in the theoretical research of chairman and general manager. According to the theory, the principal-agent relationship arises between the shareholders who hold the ownership of the company and the general manager who holds the control right of the company, and then the agency cost is generated [16]. If the chairman and the general manager are the same person, when dealing with the complex and changeable industry environment, they can give full play to the leader's spirit of risk-taking, respond quickly and efficiently, and avoid missing opportunities due to factors such as communication and consultation. Then flexible R & D decision-making, improve the performance of enterprises. Based on this, this paper proposes the following assumptions:

7

H6：If the chairman and the general manager are the same person, it may have a positive impact on the intensity of R & D investment.

2.1.7 Executive incentive

Incentive mechanism is an important content of corporate governance. Executive incentive mainly includes two aspects: equity incentive and compensation incentive. No matter which incentive mode, it is beneficial to ease the agency conflict, promote the convergence of managers' rights and interests with shareholders' rights and interests, so that executives can focus on the long-term benefits of the enterprise and have the powerful motivation to improve the technological innovation ability of the enterprise. Zahra et al. [17], Miller et al. [18] think that managers who own equity are more willing to take risks, which is beneficial to promote investment in technological innovation. Lin et al have proved that the annual salary of general manager is significant positively correlated with the intensity of investment in R & D [19]. Xu Jinfan and others pointed out that The more motivated managers are, the more motivated they are to invest in technological innovation [20]. Lu Tong et al. [5], Peng Zhong et al. [21] found that the proportion of management ownership was positive correlated with R & D investment. Liu Wei and other empirical evidence proved a significant positive correlation between executive ownership and R & D spending [22]. Based on this, this paper proposes the following assumptions:

H7a：Executive equity incentive has a positive impact on R & D investment intensity.

H7b：Executive compensation incentive has a positive impact on R & D investment intensity.

2.2 The intensity of R & D investment and enterprise performance

Innovation is the inexhaustible motive force for the development of pharmaceutical enterprises, and innovation ability is the core competitiveness of pharmaceutical enterprises. Most of the previous studies showed that there was a significant positive correlation between R & D investment intensity and corporate performance. Many found that R & D investment promoted the growth of sales revenue and corporate performance. And the greater the R & D intensity, the faster the performance improvement [23]. Johnson & Pazderka points out that the fundamental purpose of R & D investment is to gain competitive advantage that is different from other enterprises by enhancing the innovation ability of the enterprise. Ultimately improving performance [24] .Aghion et al.'s findings are the same as those of Aghion et al. Aboody et al pointed out that by increasing R & D investment, enterprises can introduce innovative products, improve technological processes, and ultimately significantly improve performance. Jefferson et al., through empirical estimates, found that the rate of return on R & D expenditure is much higher than the rate of return on fixed asset investment [27]. Chinese scholars have also carried out a lot of research work (Wu Yanbing et al., 2011 [28], Lu Guoqing et al., 2011 [29], Zhang Qixiu et al., 2012 [12], Wu Xiang, 2015 [14], Li Wei et al., 2016 [30]), they all confirmed the positive effect of R & D investment intensity on enterprise performance.

According to Enterprise Accounting Standard No. 6-Intangible assets, the expenditure in the research stage is all included in the current profit and loss when it occurs, and the expenditure in the development stage can recognize as intangible assets only when certain conditions met. Therefore, R & D investment has the characteristics of profit lag, that is, increasing R & D investment may have a negative impact on current performance, while R & D success will have a positive impact on long-term performance. This lag effect will increase the uncertainty of the innovation process, thus affecting the allocation of innovation resources and economic benefits of enterprises [31]. Based on this, this paper proposes the following assumptions:

H8: The current R & D investment intensity has a negative impact on the current performance and a positive impact on the long-term performance.

3. Test models, research samples and data

3.1 Sample selection and data sources

In this paper, choose the main board of Shanghai and Shenzhen, small and medium-sized enterprises board and gem selected listed enterprises in the pharmaceutical industry as the research objects. The selected samples include 66 Shanghai and Shenzhen main board enterprises, 43 small and medium-sized board enterprises, 24 gem enterprises, and a total of 133 enterprises. After removing ST enterprises and data missing enterprises, the selected sample includes 66 Shanghai and Shenzhen main board enterprises, 43 small and medium-sized board enterprises and 24 gem enterprises. A total of 1064 sets of effective observations from 2009 to 2016 were selected to analyze the balance panel data of sample enterprises. Corporate equity nature and R & D investment intensity data are chosen from Juchao Information Network; other data is chosen from the CSMAR database. The data analysis software is STATA 13.0.

3.2 Variable definition and Model Construction

The definitions of specific variables are shown in Table 1.

Table 1 variable definition

Name	Symbol	Computational method
Enterprise performance	ROA	Net profit / average balance of total assets
investment intensity	RD	R & D input / operating income
Nature of stock rights	STATE	Virtual variable, state = 1, non-state = 0
Equity concentration	TOP1	Number of shares held by the largest shareholder / total number of shares
Equity balance degree	ERR	Sum of shares held by the second to tenth largest shareholders / proportion of the largest shareholders
Board size	BS	Number of boards of directors
Proportion of independent directors	INDEP	Number of independent directors / board of directors
Two-job setup	DUAL	Virtual variable, both jobs = 1, other = 0
Executive equity incentive	EXI	Number of executive shares held / total number of shares
Executive compensation incentive	LNPAY	Total compensation of the top three executives taken natural logarithm
Company size	SIZE	Natural logarithm of total assets
Asset-liability ratio	LEV	Total liabilities / total assets
Increase rate of business revenue	GROWTH	(operating income for the current period-year-on-year amount) / amount for the same period of last year

First, this paper discusses the relationship between the factors of corporate governance structure and the intensity of R & D investment in pharmaceutical enterprises. The multivariate linear regression model constructed as follows:

$$RD = \beta_0 + \gamma_n * CG_n + \beta_1 * SIZE + \beta_2 * LEV + \beta_3 * GROWTH + \varepsilon$$

（1）

11

Among them, n=1、2、3、4、5、6、7、8，$CG_1 \sim CG_8$ represent the nature of equity, equity concentration, equity balance, board size, proportion of independent directors, two positions, executive equity incentives, executive compensation incentives. $\gamma_1 \sim \gamma_8$ are the corresponding coefficient.

Next, we test the lag effect of R & D investment intensity on performance, and construct the multiple linear regression model as follows:

$$ROA_k = \alpha_0 + \alpha_1 * RD + \alpha_2 * SIZE + \alpha_3 * LEV + \alpha_4 * GROWTH + \varepsilon$$

（2）

Of which K is used to denote the number of lag years. K=0 means no lag, K=1 means one year lag, and so on.

3.3 Descriptive statistics of variables

Table 2 reports descriptive statistical results for major variables.

Table 2 descriptive statistics of major variables

Variable	minimum value	maximum value	average value	mean deviation
ROA	-0.286	0.464	0.069	0.062
RD	0.170	52.610	4.375	3.475
STATE	0.000	1.000	0.323	0.468
TOP1	3.890	71.560	34.216	14.306
ERR	0.080	4.538	0.894	0.731
DUAL	0.000	1.000	0.279	0.449
INDEP	0.250	0.625	0.367	0.051
BS	5.000	15.000	8.820	1.562
EXI	0.000	25.998	15.355	10.970
LNPAY	-0.633	16.000	4.887	6.517
SIZE	12.499	25.133	17.021	3.973
LEV	0.000	9.613	0.170	0.391
GROWTH	-0.861	2.251	0.276	0.234

According to the table, the average R & D investment intensity of pharmaceutical listed enterprises in China is 4.38%, which is higher than 2.12% of the national R & D investment intensity in 2017. However, there is still a big gap from the average of 18.04 percent for the top 10 global drug companies invested in research and development in fiscal year 2015-2016. And, domestic high R & D investment

12

intensity and low R & D investment intensity of pharmaceutical enterprises, there is also a big gap.

At the level of corporate governance, 133 pharmaceutical enterprises in China have 43 holding companies and 90 non-state-owned enterprises, the distribution of equity concentration is very uneven, the distribution of equity balance degree is relatively balanced, and the distribution of equity balance degree is relatively balanced. There are 37 enterprises with two positions of chairman and general manager, and 96 enterprises with non-two positions. The board of directors has at least 5 people, up to 15, with an average of 8 people, in which the proportion of independent directors accounts for 1~3. There is a large gap between the scale of different enterprises, the equity incentive and salary incentive for the senior executives, and the difference of the ratio of assets to liabilities and the growth rate of operating income is relatively small.

3.4 Correlation analysis of variables

Table 3 reports the results of the correlation analysis of the main variables

Table 3 correlation analysis of main variables

variable	ROA	RD	STATE	TOP1	ZI	DUAL	INDEP	BS	EXI	LNPAY	SIZE	LEV	GROWTH
ROA	1.000												
RD	-0.039	1.000											
STATE	-0.164***	-0.153***	1.000										
TOP1	0.143***	-0.121***	0.050	1.000									
ZI	0.005	0.224***	-0.166***	-0.682***	1.000								
DUAL	0.019	0.207***	-0.060*	-0.087***	0.048	1.000							
INDEP	-0.089***	0.036	-0.045	0.042	-0.055*	0.053	1.000						
BS	-0.026	-0.143***	0.160***	0.114***	-0.084***	-0.180***	-0.308***	1.000					
EXI	0.108***	-0.053	-0.040	-0.030	0.007	0.017	0.041	-0.064**	1.000				
LNPAY	-0.080**	0.043	0.044	0.042	-0.005	-0.012	-0.045	0.084***	-0.991***	1.000			
SIZE	-0.080**	0.079**	0.075**	0.063**	-0.050	-0.036	-0.040	0.102***	-0.972***	0.976***	1.000		
LEV	-0.020	0.164***	-0.029	0.013	-0.008	0.133***	0.006	0.016	-0.291***	0.289***	0.289***	1.000	
GROWTH	-0.096***	-0.140***	0.122***	-0.056*	-0.032	0.040	-0.014	0.085***	0.307***	-0.293***	-0.286***	-0.155***	1.000

Note: *, **, *** are statistically significant at 10%, 5%, and 1%, respectively.

According to the results of correlation analysis, most of the variables of corporate governance structure are significant related to the intensity of R & D investment, and there is a negative relationship between R & D investment intensity and performance in the same period, which provides preliminary evidence for the verification of assumptions.

4. Empirical results

4.1 Corporate governance structure and R & D investment intensity

The regression results between the variables of corporate governance structure and the intensity of R & D investment are shown in Table 4.

Table 4 regression results of corporate governance structure and R & D investment intensity

Variable	Model 1 RD	Model 2 RD	Model 3 RD	Model 4 RD
STATE	-0.603**	-0.672**		
	(-2.070)	(-2.270)		
TOP1	0.009	0.003		
	(0.700)	(0.250)		
ERR	1.169***	1.014***		
	(4.670)	(4.010)		
DUAL	1.459***		1.372***	
	(5.010)		(4.580)	
INDEP	0.105		0.525	
	(0.040)		(0.190)	
BS	-0.229**		-0.243***	
	(-2.470)		(-2.630)	
EXI	0.001			-0.045
	(0.010)			(-0.520)
LNPAY	-0.426***			-0.375**
	(-2.890)			(-2.490)
SIZE	0.772***	0.045	0.130**	0.565***
	(4.850)	(0.880)	(2.250)	(3.510)
LEV	0.981***	1.207***	1.025***	1.427***
	(3.130)	(3.830)	(3.180)	(4.470)
GROWTH	-1.221*	-1.394**	-1.769***	-1.792***
	(-1.820)	(-2.130)	(-2.700)	(-2.780)
Constant	-5.982*	3.155***	4.412**	-2.193
	(-1.710)	(3.130)	(2.480)	(-0.650)
N	1064	1064	1064	1064
R^2	0.166	0.096	0.094	0.061
Adjust R^2	0.153	0.088	0.087	0.055
F	12.640	12.860	12.310	9.430
P	0.000	0.000	0.000	0.000

Note: Dependent variable: RD. The bracketed values are t; *, **, *** are significant at the 10%, 5%, 1% statistical levels, respectively.

16

Model 1 is a full sample regression of the intensity of R & D investment by eight variables of corporate governance structure; Model 2~4 divides the corporate governance structure into equity structure, board governance and executive incentive to return to the intensity of R & D investment respectively. The regression results were consistent. Firstly, in terms of ownership structure, state-owned holding negatively correlated with R & D investment intensity at 5% level, H1 is established, and equity concentration has a positive effect on R & D investment intensity, but it is not significant, H2 is established; Equity balance at the level of 1% significantly positive impact on R & D investment intensity, H3 is established. In the governance of the board of directors, the chairperson and the both positions of general manager and general manager have a positive effect on R & D investment intensity at a significant level of 1%, H4 is established, and the proportion of independent directors is positive. However, not significant, H5 is established; the size of the board of directors negatively correlated with the intensity of R & D investment. That is, the larger the board size, the larger the number of people, and the more unfavorable the R & D investment, H6 is established. In executive incentive, equity incentive has no significant effect on R & D investment intensity, and the direction is not clear, H7a is not valid, compensation incentive has a significant negative impact, H7b is not valid. In terms of controlling variables, the size of the company and the ratio of assets to liabilities have a significant positive impact on the intensity of investment in R & D; the growth rate showed a negative and significant effect.

4.2 The intensity of R & D investment and enterprise performance

The regression between R & D investment intensity and enterprise performance (ROA) is shown in Table 5.

Table 5 regression results between R & D input intensity and Enterprise performance (ROA)

Variable	Model 5 ROA	Model 6 ROA_1	Model 7 ROA_2	Model 8 ROA_3	Model 9 ROA_4	Model 10 ROA_5	Model 11 ROA_6	Model 12 ROA_7
RD	-0.001**	-0.001	0.001	0.001	0.002**	0.001*	0.002***	0.006***
	(-2.240)	(-1.030)	(1.180)	(0.860)	(2.470)	(1.940)	(2.670)	(3.170)
SIZE	-0.001	0.002**	0.005***	0.021***	0.018***	0.012***	0.015***	0.017**
	(-1.080)	(2.150)	(3.950)	(6.830)	(5.040)	(3.320)	(3.330)	(2.400)
LEV	0.010*	0.014***	0.018***	0.029***	0.016	0.016	-0.015	-0.070
	(1.750)	(2.660)	(3.410)	(5.790)	(1.140)	(0.920)	(-0.460)	(-1.150)
GROWT H	-0.063***	-0.092***	-0.115***	-0.119***	-0.121***	-0.118***	-0.119***	-0.115***
	(-5.600)	(-8.410)	(-9.930)	(-10.430)	(-9.070)	(-8.440)	(-6.740)	(-4.230)
Constant	0.113***	0.075***	0.026	-0.198***	-0.154***	-0.082	-0.121*	-0.170*
	(7.540)	(5.040)	(1.280)	(-4.450)	(-3.030)	(-1.520)	(-1.860)	(-1.670)
R^2	0.049	0.118	0.192	0.276	0.238	0.245	0.281	0.363
Adjust R^2	0.044	0.113	0.187	0.271	0.231	0.236	0.267	0.334
F	9.380	23.830	38.650	55.880	35.690	26.420	19.670	12.420
P	0.000	0.000	0.000	0.000	0.000	0.000	0.000	0.000

Note: dependent variable: ROA. The bracketed values are t; *, **, *** are significant at 10%, 5%, and 1% statistical levels, respectively.

Model 5 is the regression of R & D investment intensity of enterprise performance in the same year, while model 6~12 is 1, 2, 3, 4, 5, 6, 7 years later. First, in the same year, R & D investment intensity is negatively correlated with enterprise performance at a significant level of 5%, while one year later, it will still be negatively correlated with R & D investment intensity, but not significant. There is no significant positive correlation between R & D investment intensity and performance of 2 years behind. 3 years later, the performance will not be significant correlated with R & D investment intensity. 4~5 years later, the performance will be positive correlated with R & D investment intensity of 5% and 10%, 6 years behind and 1% ,7 years behind. The regression results show that the current R & D investment intensity has a negative

18

impact on the current performance. With the passage of time, the R & D investment intensity gradually changes from a negative to a positive impact, and the positive impact is more and more significant. H8 is established.

5. Robustness test

In this paper, ROE (net profit / average balance of shareholders' equity) is selected to measure the performance of enterprises, and the lag effect of R & D investment intensity on performance is tested. The regression results are shown in Table 6.

Table 6 regression results of R & D Investment intensity on Enterprise performance (ROE)

Variable	Mode 13	Mode 14	Mode 15	Mode 16	Mode 17	Mode 18	Mode 19	Mode 20
	ROE	ROE_1	ROE_2	ROE_3	ROE_4	ROE_5	ROE_6	ROE_7
RD	-0.004***	-0.002*	0.001	0.0004	0.003	0.002	0.002**	0.009**
	(-3.350)	(-1.850)	(0.540)	(0.300)	(1.640)	(1.340)	(1.990)	(2.650)
SIZE	-0.002	0.003*	0.007**	0.037***	0.031***	0.019***	0.022***	0.023*
	(-1.320)	(1.790)	(2.500)	(4.960)	(3.360)	(2.760)	(3.090)	(1.920)
LEV	0.014	0.016*	0.031***	0.035***	0.033	-0.056*	-0.128**	-0.274**
	(1.510)	(1.850)	(2.660)	(2.940)	(0.900)	(-1.670)	(-2.330)	(-2.650)
GROWTH	-0.082***	-0.131***	-0.096***	-0.140***	-0.094***	-0.107***	-0.105***	-0.124***
	(-4.500)	(-7.320)	(-3.800)	(-5.100)	(-2.720)	(-4.030)	(-3.650)	(-2.700)
Constant	0.169***	0.107***	0.017	-0.391***	-0.331**	-0.164	-0.206*	-0.231
	(6.900)	(4.360)	(0.370)	(-3.650)	(-2.500)	(-1.600)	(-1.940)	(-1.340)
R^2	0.040	0.088	0.051	0.105	0.060	0.095	0.160	0.264
Adjust R^2	0.035	0.083	0.045	0.099	0.052	0.084	0.143	0.230
F	7.680	17.220	8.780	17.260	7.270	8.500	9.580	7.800
P	0.000	0.000	0.000	0.000	0.000	0.000	0.000	0.000

Note: dependent variable: ROE. The bracketed values are t; *, **, ***are significant at 10%, 5%, and 1% statistical levels, respectively.

Model 13 is the regression of enterprise performance to R & D investment intensity in the same year, and model 14~20 is the regression of R & D investment intensity after 1, 2, 3, 4, 5, 6, 7 years of performance. The regression results show that with the passage of time, the relationship between the two changes from significant negative to significant positive, which proves the robustness of the above conclusion.

6. Conclusion and suggestion

According to the empirical analysis of the intensity of R & D investment by corporate governance structure, first, in terms of equity structure, state-owned holding does have a negative impact on the intensity of R & D investment compared with non-state-owned holding. Therefore, we should continue to promote the reform of mixed ownership of state-owned enterprises, introduce the market-oriented mechanism, optimize the governance structure, promote it to increase R & D investment, and focus on enhancing the efficiency of R & D investment into performance. At the same time, considering the higher R & D input intensity of the non-state-owned holding enterprises, it suggests that the allocation of innovation resources should tilted towards the non-state-owned holding enterprises. The positive effect of equity concentration on the intensity of R & D investment reflects the major shareholders of the enterprise. Pay attention to long-term development, dare to take risks, thus effectively stimulate the enterprise's innovative R & D activities. The significant positive effect of equity balance degree shows that the introduction of checks and balances system among large shareholders can effectively reduce agency conflicts, guarantee the scientific decision-making, and then improve the efficiency of R & D investment transforming into enterprise performance. In the governance of the board of directors, if the chairman and the general manager are the same person, he or she will be conducive to his or her full play of the spirit of risk-taking, the rapid and efficient formulation of R & D strategy, in a competitive market in an invincible position. The addition of independent directors can open up the enterprise's vision, fully absorb the opinions and suggestions from the outside, and be conducive to improving the quality of decision-making and promoting innovation. R & D process. However, the role of independent directors is not significant, and the independent director system needs to be further improved. Rewards and punishments can be set up to promote independent directors to enhance their sense of responsibility and play a due role in supervision. The expansion of board size leads to inefficient management, poor communication and lower decision-making efficiency. It suggests that companies gradually explore the most efficient board size, introduce board members that are more capable or abolish board members who cannot play their due role. In terms of executive incentives, equity incentives and compensation incentives do not play a significant positive role in R & D as expected, which means they do not prompt executives to promote R & D strategy and improve investment in R & D. Therefore, the incentive mechanism of pharmaceutical companies to senior executives needs to be further improved, in order to improve the sensitivity of executive pay performance and make them focus on innovative R & D decisions, which are in line with the long-term interests of enterprises.

According to the test results of the influence of R & D investment intensity on enterprise performance lag effect, we can see that with the passage of time, the relationship between R & D investment and R & D investment gradually changes from significant negative to significant positive, but the duration is longer. That is to say, the efficiency of innovation R & D investment into enterprise performance still needs to improve largely. It suggests that the whole process of new drug research and development should be considered, and the resources of innovation should reasonably allocate. Since new drug research and development needs to go through many links, and the requirements for technological innovation ability are different in each link, we can determine the appropriate weight to allocate the innovation resources reasonably through comprehensive evaluation. Second, we should follow the rules of technological innovation of pharmaceutical enterprises, and keep absorbing, learning and creating new technologies and processes, manage innovation activities efficiently, improve R & D efficiency. Finally, domestic pharmaceutical enterprises are weak in basic research, it suggests integrating and utilizing internal and external resources. Internal, we can fully integrate the strength of universities and professional research institutions. Overseas, we can strengthen cooperation with multinational pharmaceutical enterprises, while learning advanced technology and management experience. We can constantly improve our own strength, and strive to promote the process of localization innovation.

7. References

[1] The 13th five-year Plan of Pharmaceutical Industry will focus on promoting innovation [J]. Journal of China Pharmaceutical University, 2015, 46 (06): 658.

[2] Li Shengkun, Zhang Anqi. Corporate Governance, technological Innovation and Corporate performance-an empirical study based on the data of listed companies in Henan Province [J]. Friends of Accounting, 2016 (24): 99-103.

[3] Xiang chaojin,Xie Ming. Empirical Analysis on the relationship between listed Company performance and Corporate Governance structure in China [J]. Managing the World, 2003 (05): 117-124.

[4] Zhou Jian, Wang Pengfei, Li Wenjia, Chen Surong. Research on the relationship between Corporate Governance structure and performance of innovative Enterprises-based on empirical evidence of listed companies on gem [J]. Economic and Management Research, 2012 (04): 106-115.

[5] Lu Tong, party seal. Corporate governance and technological innovation: sub-industry comparison [J]. Economic Research, 2014, 49 (06): 115-128.

[6] Chen Lilin, Feng Xingyu. Based on the governance structure of IT industry, the research on the relationship between R D investment and enterprise performance [J]. Research and Development Management, 2015, 27 (03): 45-56.

[7] Ye Chen Gang, Qiu Li, Zhang Lijuan. Corporate governance structure, internal control quality and corporate financial performance [J]. Audit study, 2016 (02): 104-112.

[8] Feng Taozhu, Zhang Yang, Zhang GE. Research on the influence of governance structure of listed companies on performance-based on unbalanced panel data of coal industry [J]. China Coal, 2017, 43 (06): 11-16 21.

[9] Zhang Min, Lin Ai Mei, Wei Linxin. Internal control, corporate governance structure and corporate financial performance [J]. Accounting Newsletter, 2017 (21): 75-79 129.

[10] Xie Haijuan, Liu Xiaozhen. How corporate governance affects corporate profitability-an empirical analysis of regulatory effects based on internal control intermediaries [J]. Monthly Financial and Accounting Journal, 2018 (02): 94-104.

[11] Kornai J, Weibull J W. Paternalism, buyers' and sellers' markets [J]. Mathematical

and Social Sciences, 1983, 6(2): 153-169.

[12] Zhang Qixiu, ran Yi, Chen Shou Ming, Wang Gui. Investment in R & D and Corporate performance: equity checks and balances or Equity concentration?-an empirical study based on State-owned listed companies [J]. Science of Science and Technology Management, 2012, 33 (07): 126-132.

[13] Chen Yuying, Chu Shuzhen. The influence of the governance structure of pharmaceutical listed companies on technological innovation [J]. Chinese Journal of New drugs, 2015, 24 (03): 250-254.

[14] Wu Xiang. Corporate governance, R & D investment and corporate performance [J]. Accounting Newsletter, 2017 (30): 32-36.

[15] Chen Kunyu. Innovative activities, ownership structure and operating performance of innovative enterprises-empirical evidence from A-share market in China [J]. Research on Industrial economy, 2010 (04): 49-57.

[16] Xie jie.Chairman and General Manager: the separation and unity of the two positions [J]. Finance and economy, 2006, (08): 31-32.

[17] Zahra S A, Neubaum D O, Huse M. Entrepreneurship in medium-size companies: Exploring the effects of ownership and governance systems [J]. Journal of Management, 2000, 26(5):947-976.

[18] Miller J S, Wiseman R M, Gomez-Mejia L R. The fit between CEO compensation design and firm risk [J]. Academy of Management Journal, 2002, 45(4):745-756.

[19] LIN C, LIN P, SONG F M, et al. Managerial incentives, CEO characteristics and corporate innovation in China's private sector [J]. Journal of Comparative Economics, 2011, 39(2):176-190.

[20] Xu Jinfa, Liu. Corporate governance structure and technological innovation [J]. Scientific Research Management, 2002 (04): 11-15.

[21] Peng Zhongwen, Li, Wang Meihua. Political relevance, Corporate Governance and R & D Innovation-based on panel data from listed companies in high-end equipment manufacturing [J]. Journal of Social Science, Hunan normal University, 2015, 44 (02): 124-131.

24

[22] Liu Wei, Liu Xing. An empirical study on the impact of Executive Stock ownership on RD Expenditure-empirical evidence from A-share listed companies in 2002-2004 [J]. Science of Science and Management of Science and Technology, 2007 (10): 172-175.

[23] Morby S B. Research on the value-relevance of R&D in the computer industry [J]. Academy of Management Journal, 1988, 30:51-70.

[24] Johnson L D, Pazderka B. Firm value and investment in R&D [J]. Managerial and Decision Economics, 1993, 14(1):15-24.

[25] Aghion P, Reenen J V, Zingales L. Innovation and institutional ownership[R]. NBER Working Paper, No. 14769, 2009.

[26] Aboody D, Lev B. Information asymmetry, R&D, and insider gains [J]. Journal of Finance, 2000, 55: 2747-2766.

[27] Jefferson G H, Bai H M, Guan X J, et al. R&D performance in Chinese industry [J]. Economics of Innovation and New Technology, 2006, 15(4-5): 345-366.

[28] Wu Yanbing, Mi Zengyu. Innovation, imitation and enterprise efficiency-empirical evidence from manufacturing non-state-owned enterprises [J]. Chinese Social Sciences, 2011 (04): 77-94 222.

[29] Lu Guoqing. Research on the performance of Industrial Innovation of small and medium-sized Board listed companies in China [J]. Economic Research, 2011, 46 (02): 138-148.

[30] Li Wei, Mao Qiao Ling. An empirical study on the impact of technological innovation on corporate performance of small and medium-sized listed companies-based on the perspective of corporate governance regulation [J]. Science and Technology Management Research, 2016, 36 (06): 159-162 175.

[31] Sun Ying. Research on the relationship between corporate governance, R & D investment delay effect and enterprise performance in strategic emerging industries [J]. Progress and Countermeasures in Science and Technology, 2017, 34 (05): 66-72.

YOUR KNOWLEDGE HAS VALUE

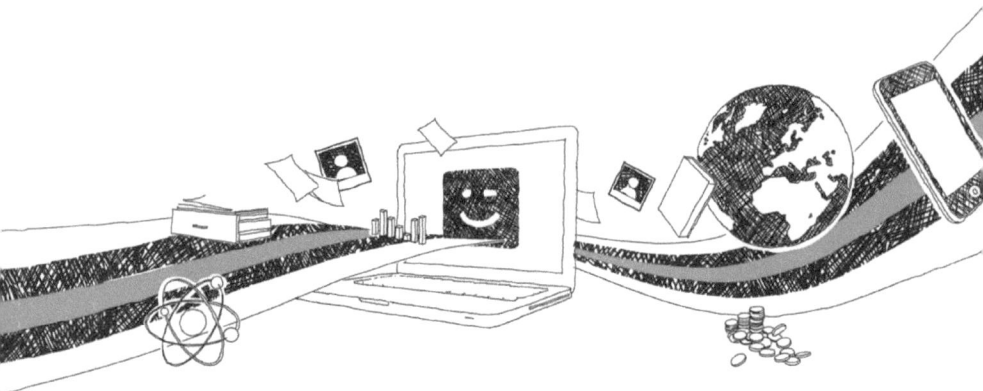